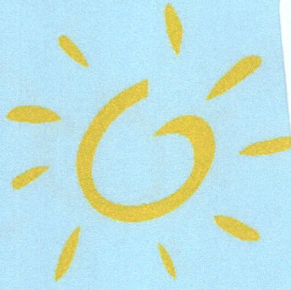

This Book Belongs to:

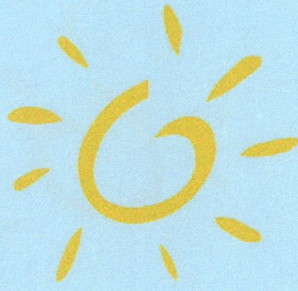

This book is dedicated to all the people who struggle daily with various kidney issues to stay alive. I am thankful you have the option of dialysis that allows you to continue to live. Keep fighting!

To all those currently waiting for a life-saving kidney, I pray you receive your gift of life soon. Keep searching, and tell everyone you know to tell everyone they know you need a kidney donor hero!

To all the donor heroes, both living and deceased, you truly are life savers and a blessing for so many. The ultimate gift of life is the greatest gift of all. As a living kidney donor, I know firsthand how amazing it feels to be able to save someone's life. So please register to be an organ donor at donatelife.net or registerme.org

Share Your Spare!

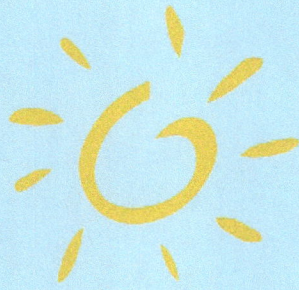

I want to extend a special thank you to my publisher and living kidney donor recipient, Mike Nicloy, for sharing your experiences about dialysis so I could better understand the process to write this book. It is no coincidence that we were brought together! I also want to thank Pat Birrenkott for sharing pictures during your dialysis to give me a visual, and to help my illustrator create a more realistic image. I pray you find your kidney donor hero soon! Thank you as well to Jeffrey Jacobson for your input about dialysis. I am so happy you have been blessed with your second kidney transplant. I pray your donor families find comfort knowing their loved one has allowed you another chance at life.

In loving memory of our Grandpa Bob who left us too soon.

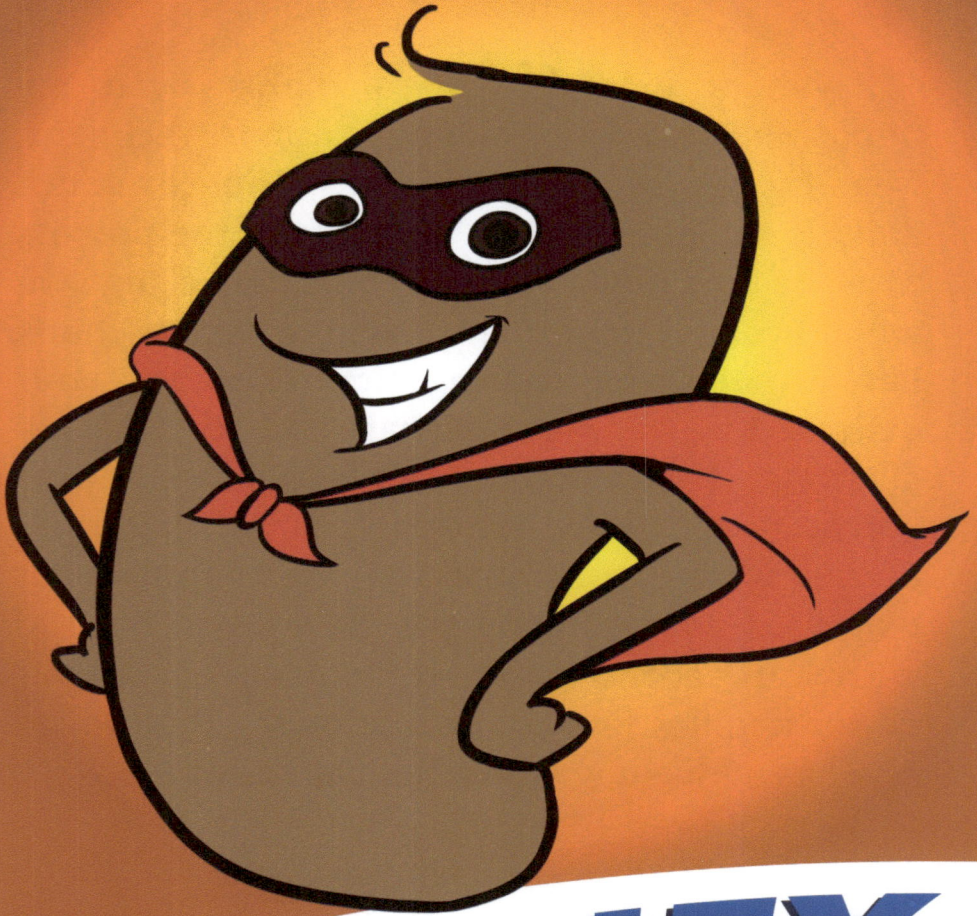

WANTED

KIDNEY HEROES

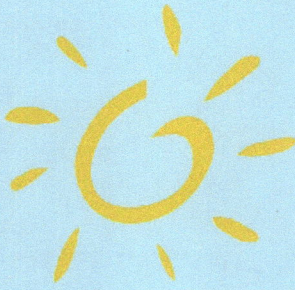

Howl and his family are familiar with organ donation because Howl received the gift of life with a heart transplant, and now Howl's Grandpa Bob is on the transplant list. He has Chronic Kidney Disease, which is also known as "CKD", and the disease makes his kidneys sick. Since Grandpa Bob's kidneys do not work the way they should, he needs a transplant to receive a new and healthy kidney. Thankfully there is a treatment available called dialysis that can do the work of the kidneys until an organ donor is hopefully found.

Thousands of owls are also waiting for a life-saving kidney, which means the wait is long and can actually be many years. Unfortunately there are many different diseases and illnesses that cause damage to the kidneys, so organ donation is especially important to help save lives.

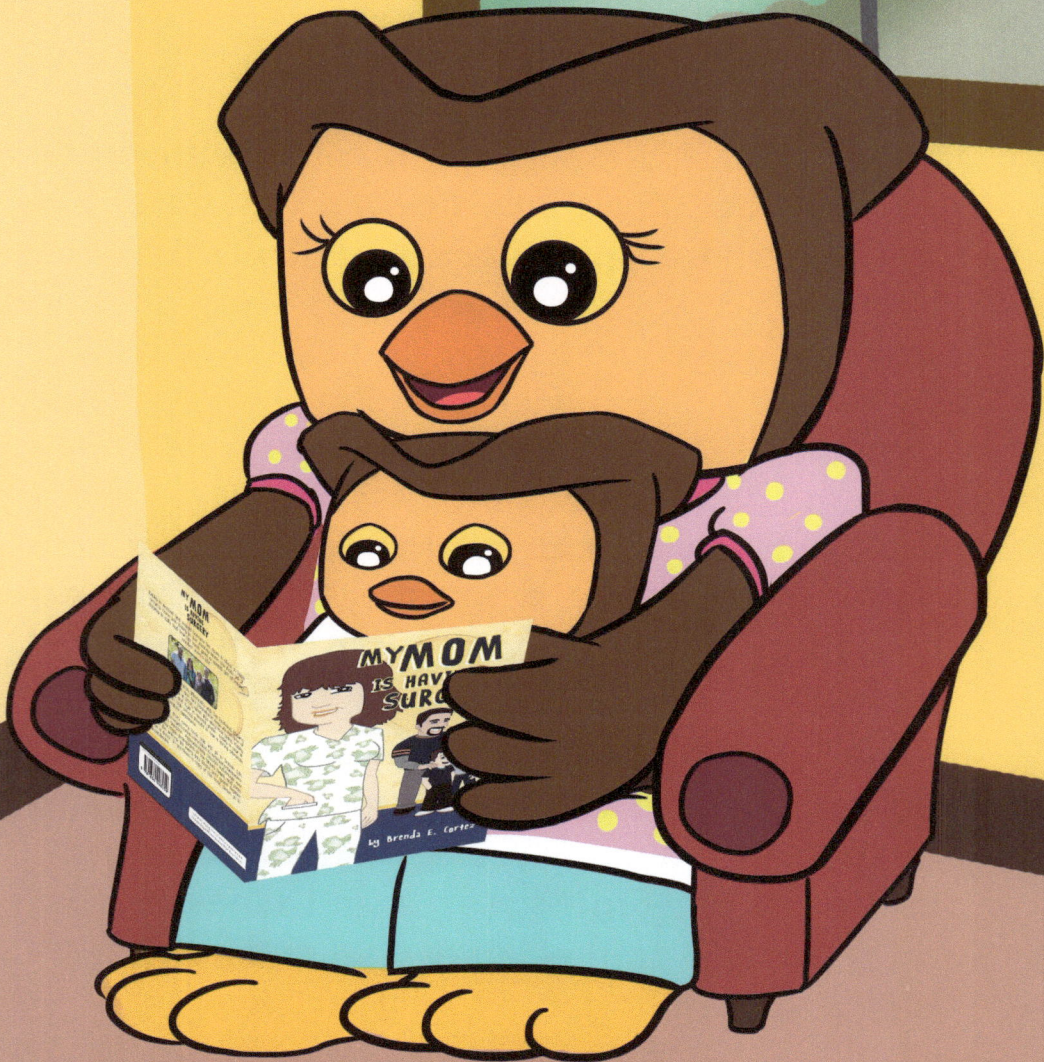

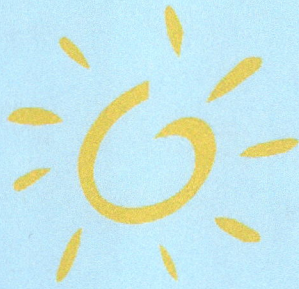

Grandpa Bob hopes to find a living donor who is willing to "share their spare" kidney. This is a saying used to promote living kidney donation because we can live with only one kidney. The other way to receive a kidney is to be added to the transplant list. This is a list of all the people who are waiting to receive a life-saving organ, and these organs come from people who have died but want to be an organ donor. If their organs are still in good condition, they want to donate them to help others live.

Howl's mom explained to him as they read a book about living kidney donation, "Organ donors are like heroes because they truly save people's lives."

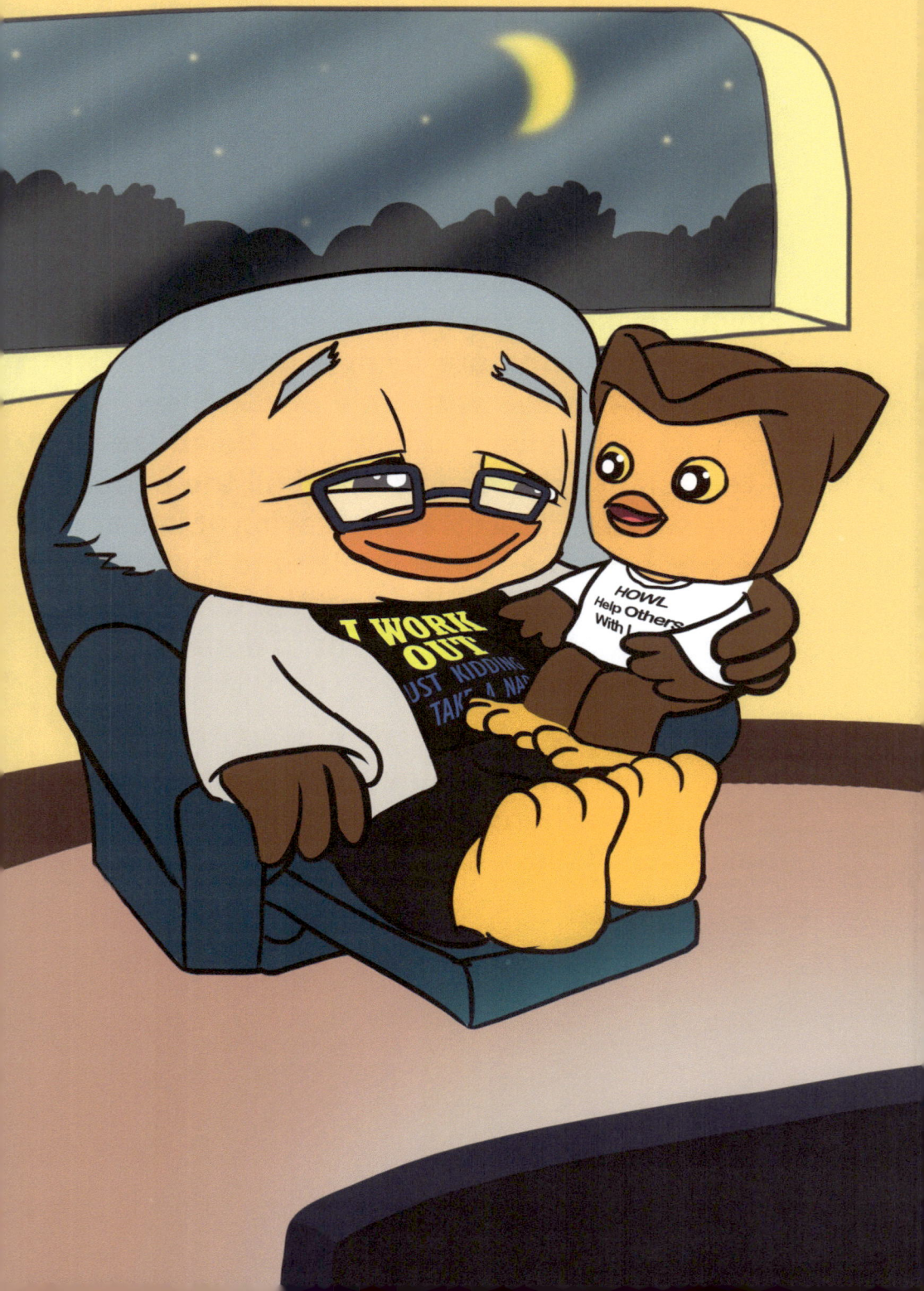

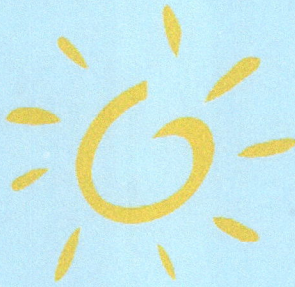

Even though Howl's Grandpa Bob is in need of a kidney, dialysis is an option that can do some of the things healthy kidneys do. Not everyone qualifies for a transplant and must depend on dialysis for the rest of their lives. Grandpa Bob does hemodialysis at a clinic, as do most patients, but some choose to do the treatment at home. Others do peritoneal dialysis which is a home based treatment.

Howl is very curious about dialysis and what it actually does. He asked Grandpa Bob, "Can I go with you to your next dialysis appointment?"

Grandpa replied, "I go every Tuesday, Thursday and Saturday, so you may come along Saturday."

Howl is excited to spend time with his grandpa because he has a lot of questions. He wants to help Grandpa Bob while at dialysis because after all, Howl stands for Help Others With Love, and he especially likes helping his grandpa.

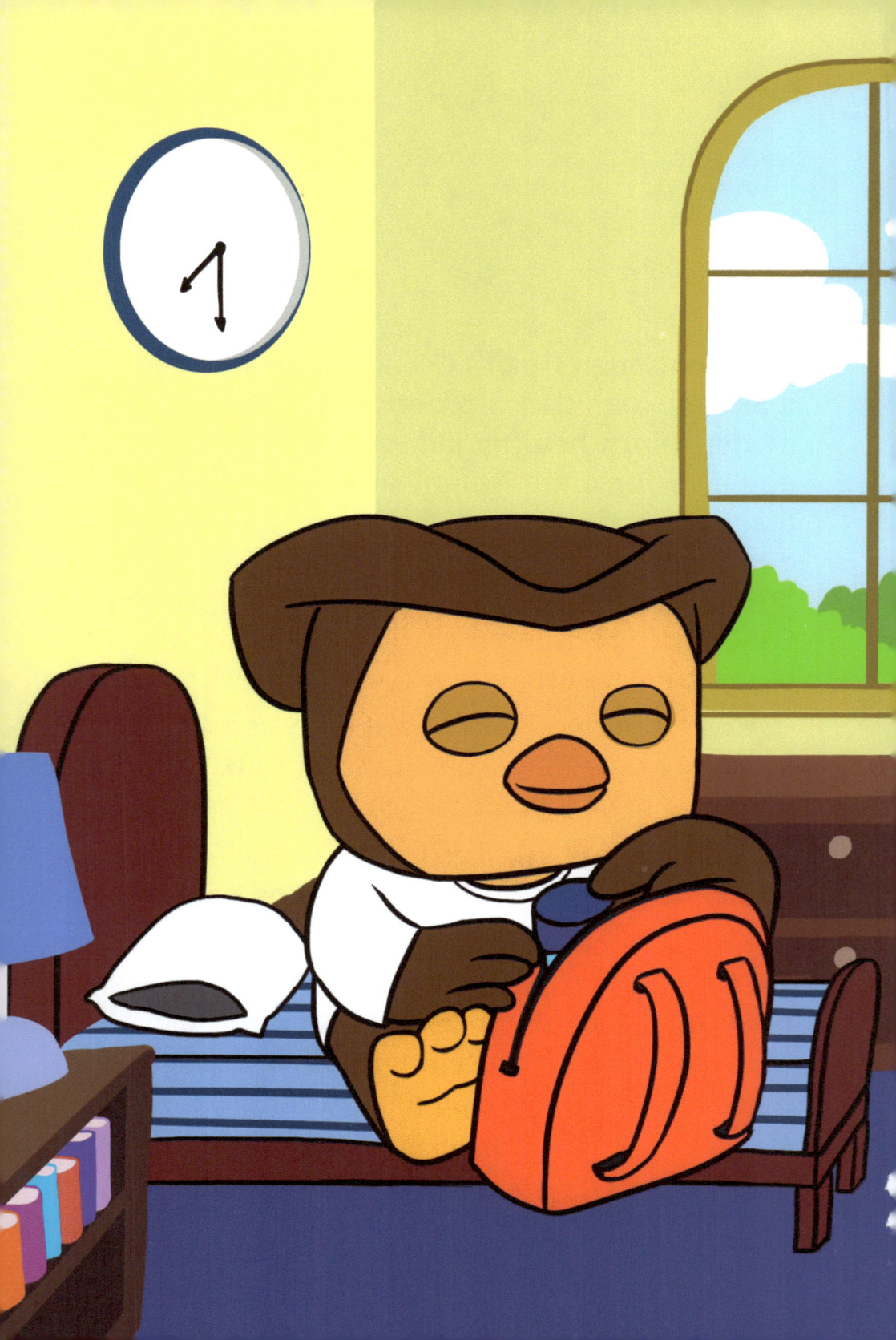

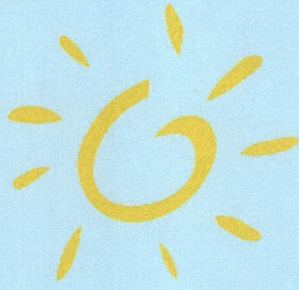

Today is Saturday, and Howl is awake bright and early. He is anxious to get to the dialysis center, and his backpack is already packed.

"Let's go, Howl, I have to be to dialysis by 9:00," announced Grandpa Bob.

"Okay Grandpa, I'm ready! How long will we be there?" Howl asked.

"My treatment takes three hours, but your dad will come get you after an hour because that can be a long time to sit and be quiet," Grandpa Bob replied.

"Why do we have to be quiet?" inquired Howl.

"So others can relax, watch TV, or sleep if they want to. Some people choose to ride the Stationary bike so they can get exercise, but many people are too tired to ride the bike," answered Grandpa Bob.

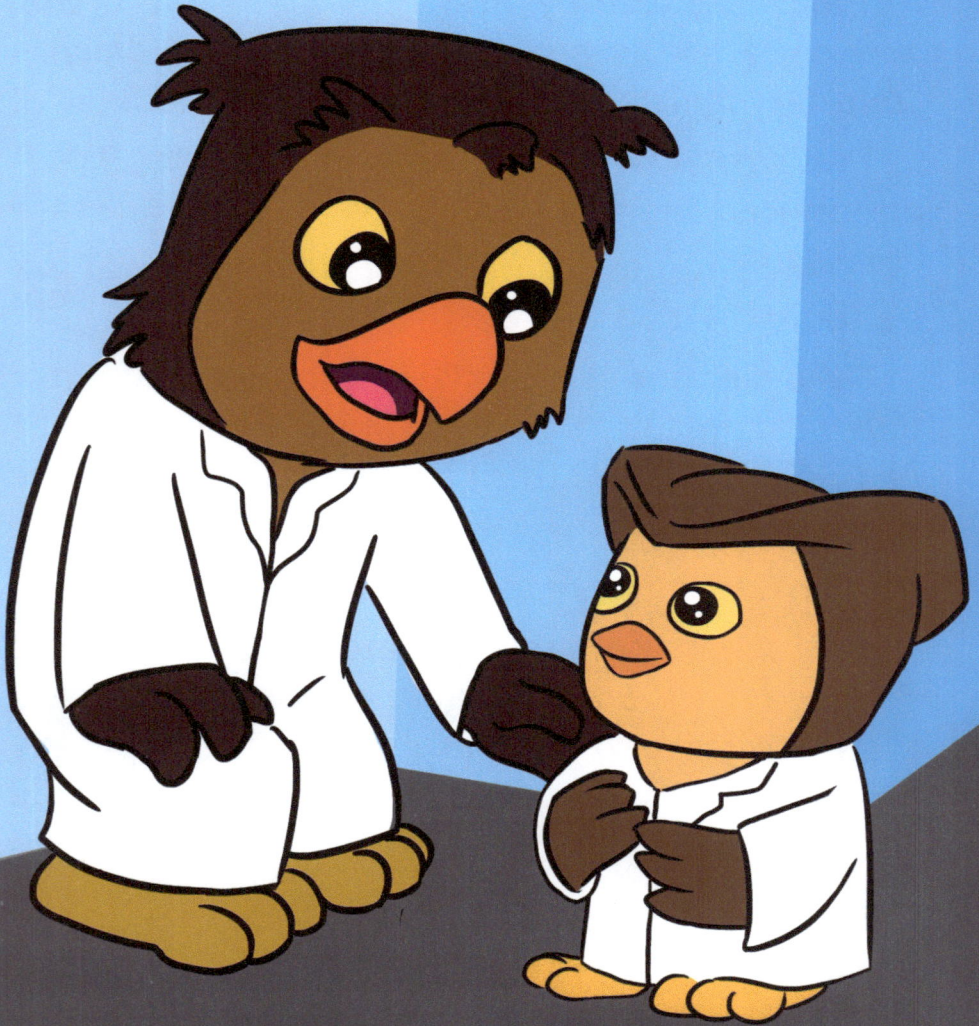

DIALYSIS
CENTER

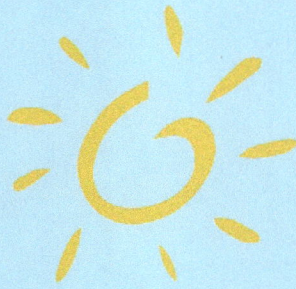

At the clinic, Howl watches as Grandpa Bob steps on the scale to be weighed, and explains how he does this at the beginning and end of every dialysis treatment. A technician, who is similar to a nurse, brings Howl to a sink to wash away any germs he may have on his hands. The technician also gives him a white lab coat to wear while he is there.

"What exactly does dialysis do?" Howl asks the technician.

"It's similar to when a car gets the oil changed. The dirty oil is drained and then replaced with clean oil," he answered. "Dialysis uses a tall machine to help take the blood out of the body, filter and clean it through the machine, and return it to the body. Many patients feel cold during their dialysis treatment, so a comfy blanket helps to warm them up."

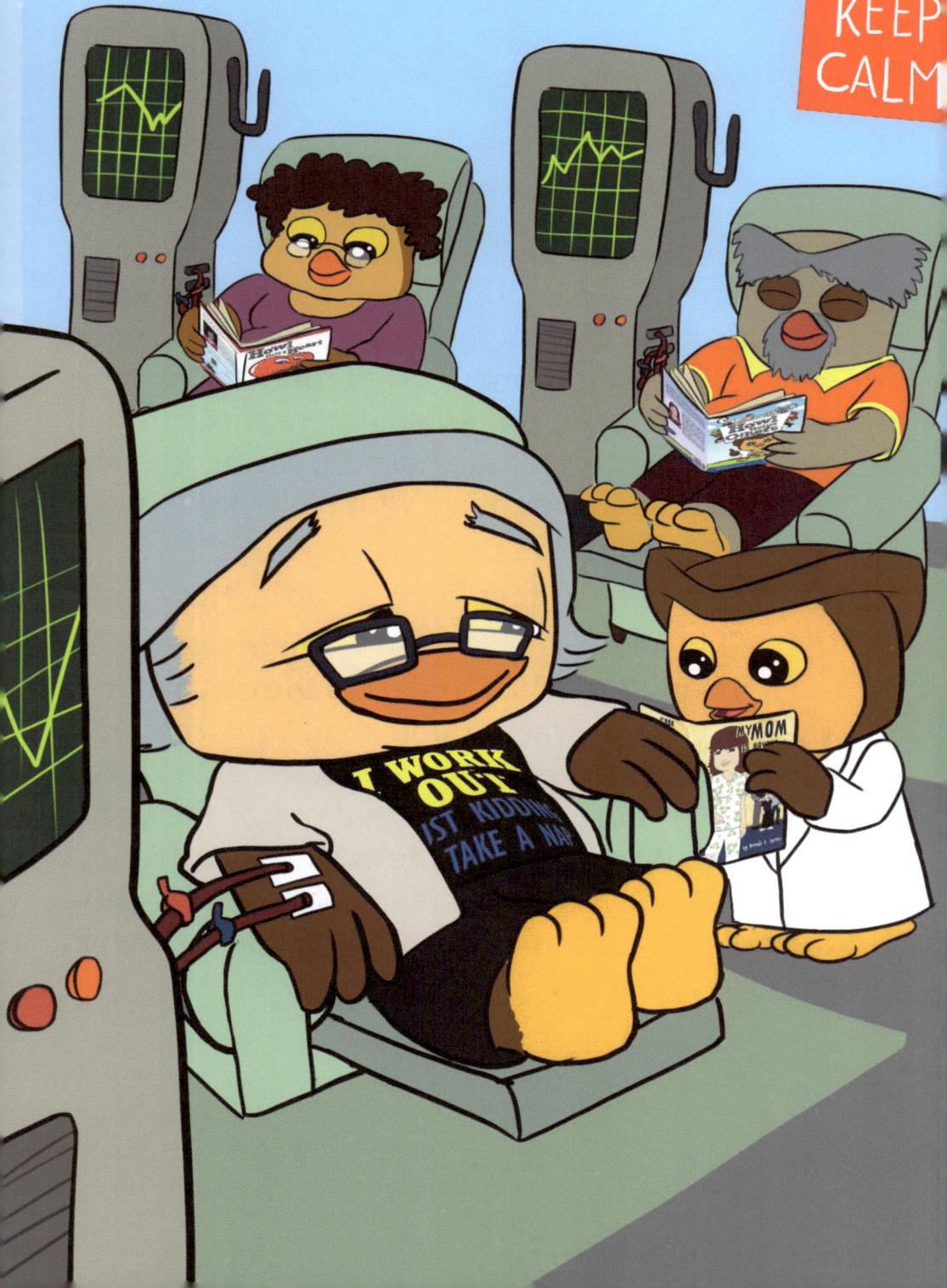

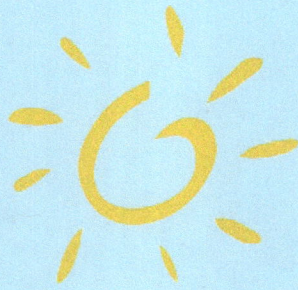

Howl nods and asks, "Where does the blood come out of and go back into the body?"

"Most of the time it is through a special port called a fistula, which is usually placed into the arm," the technician replies.

Howl and his grandpa head back to the treatment area to find a seat. The chairs are big and comfy, which is good since many of the patients sleep or read while they get their treatment. The technician comes and hooks up the machine to the fistula in grandpa's arm. A cuff is put over his other arm to check his blood pressure every 15 minutes.

Sitting quietly, Howl calmly reads his favorite book to Grandpa Bob. He looks around and notices that the other owls are either sitting calmly or sleeping. One owl looks to be close to his mom's age, and the others look older, like Grandpa Bob.

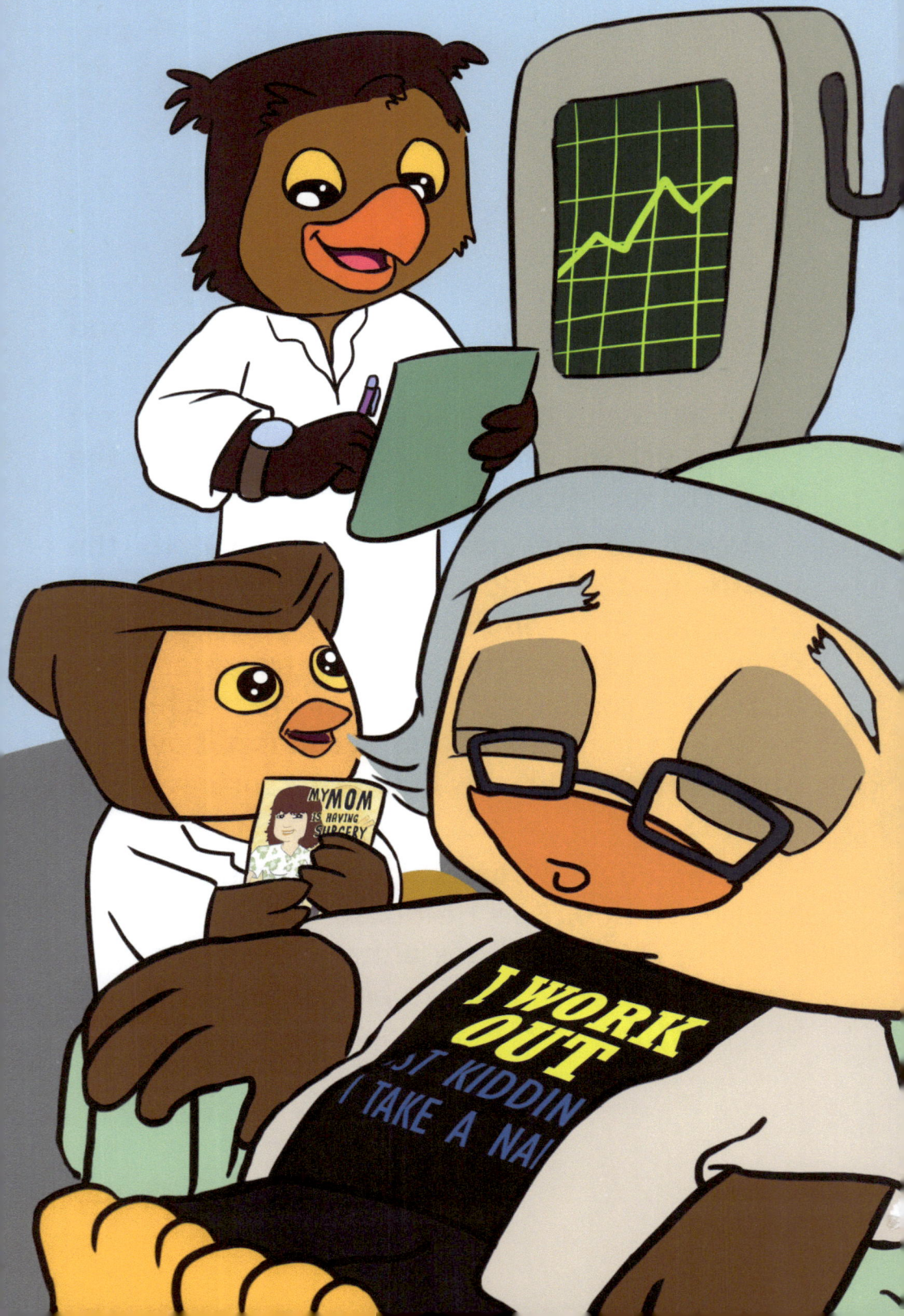

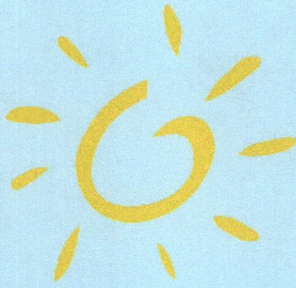

The technician comes by to check on grandpa and the machine. Grandpa has just fallen asleep, so Howl asks the technician, "Will my grandpa feel sick when he gets home?"

"He might, but everyone reacts differently" whispered the technician. "Some will be tired and hungry while others may feel fine. Your grandpa needs to make sure he doesn't drink too much water or fluids, because too many fluids can cause shortness of breath and make him feel sick."

"Thank you for explaining everything to me. I'm very glad I was able to come with Grandpa Bob to see how dialysis is keeping him alive," Howl said as he hugs the technician.

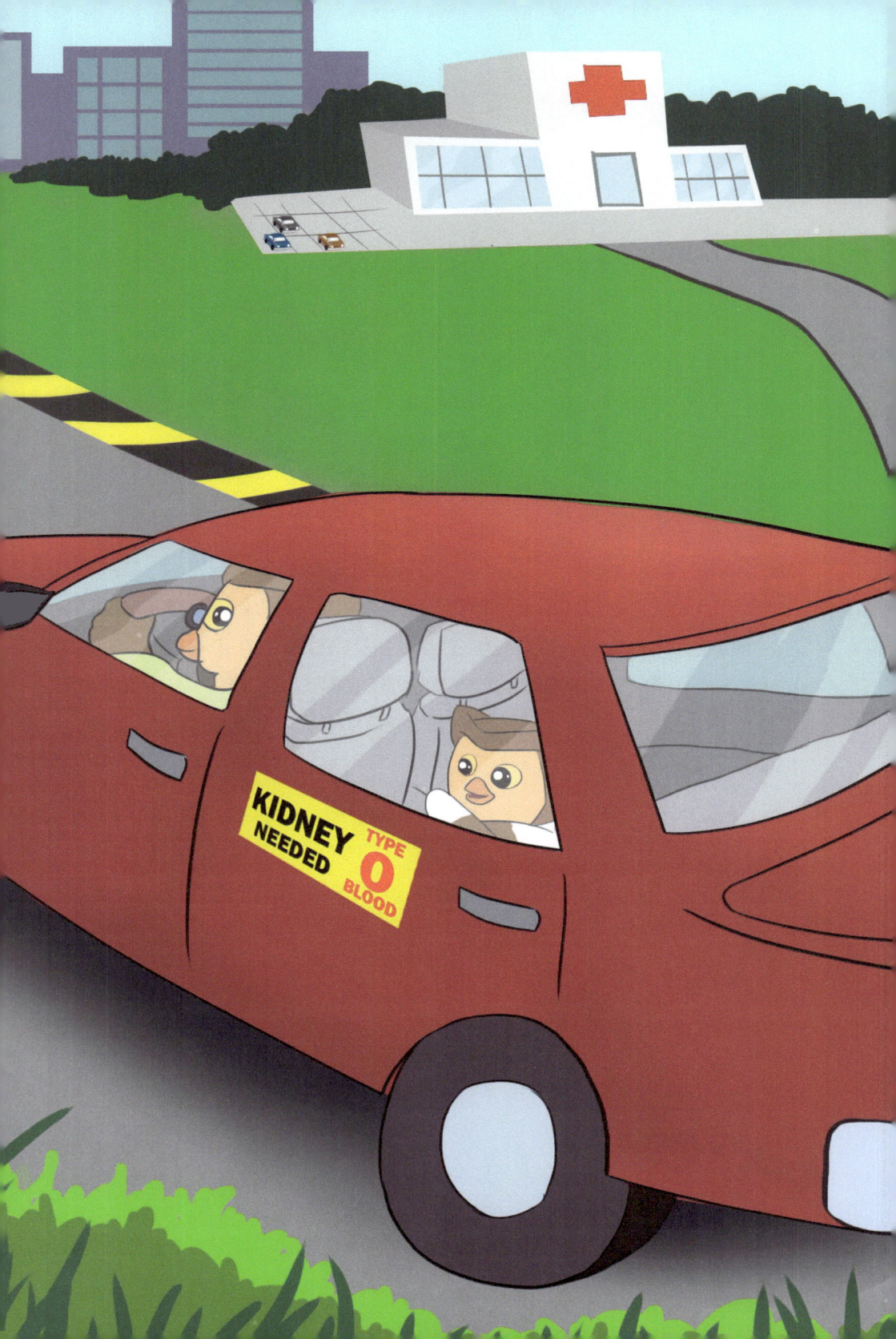

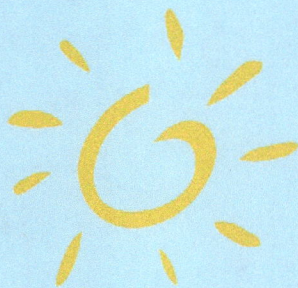

On their ride home, Howl and his dad talk about what he learned at the dialysis treatment center.

"I am so happy dialysis is helping Grandpa Bob and so many others like him who have sick kidneys," said Howl, "But dialysis doesn't seem fun at all."

"It's not," replied Howl's dad. "It takes a lot of time and is very tiring. Hopefully someday soon there will be enough available kidneys to go around for everyone in need."

"I'm happy we are helping Grandpa Bob search for his new kidney!" exclaimed Howl.

"Yes Howl, hopefully our social media posts and the sign on our car will help us find available donors," said Howl's dad.

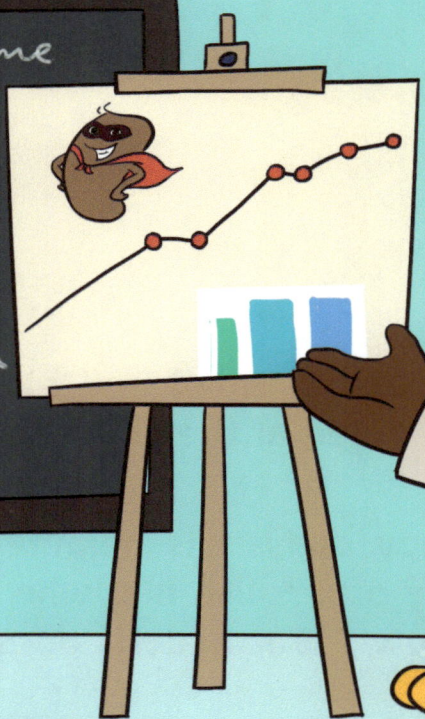

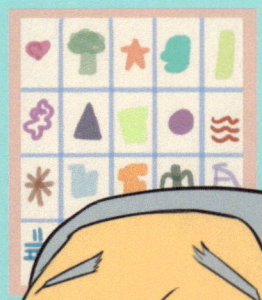

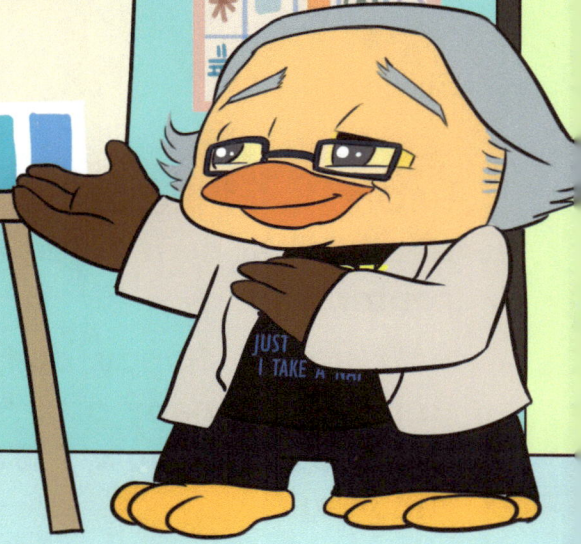

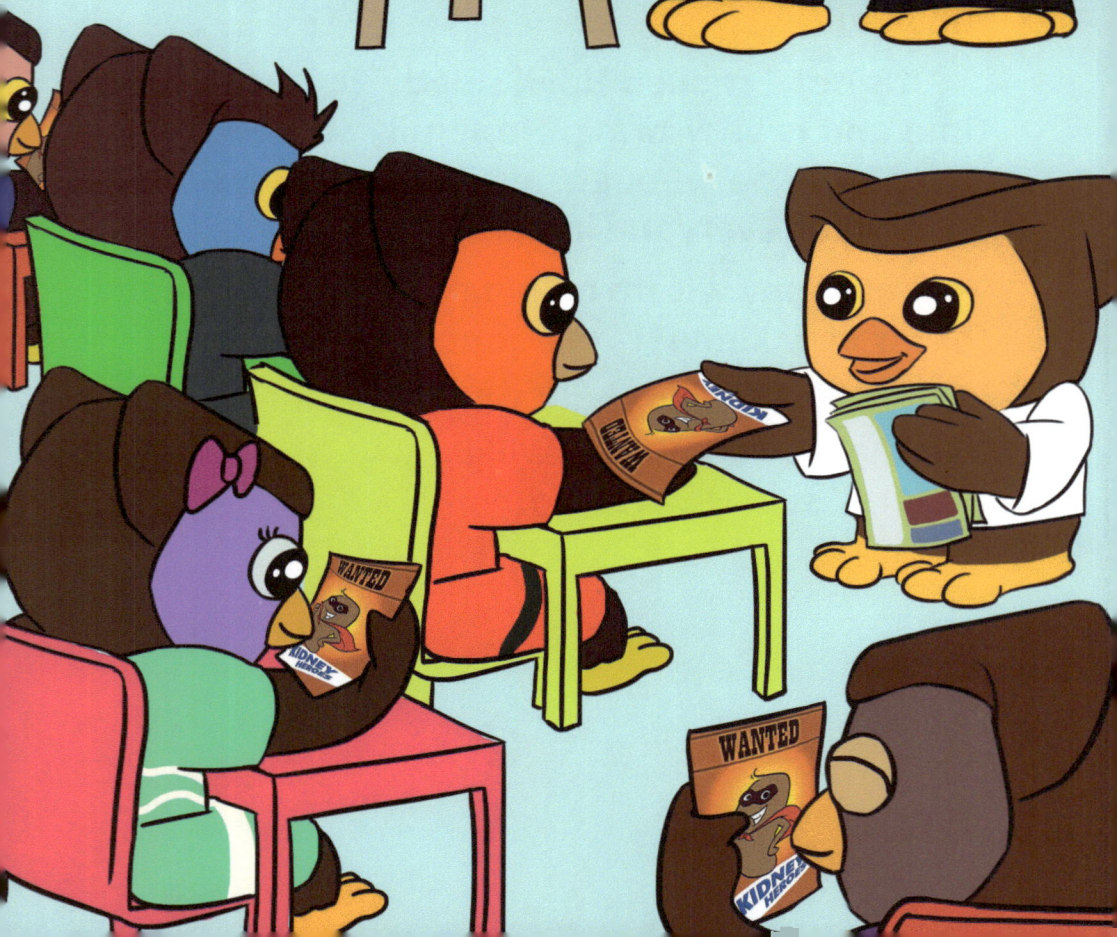

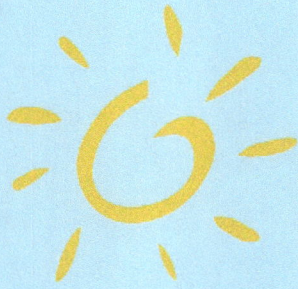

In addition to the sign on their car and social media posts, Howl and Grandpa Bob are making a presentation to Howl's class. They are teaching the class what organ donation is, how it saves lives, and that organ donors are true heroes! Grandpa Bob is explaining how many people are waiting for a life-saving organ, especially a kidney, and how living donation works.

Every student is going home with a brochure from a foundation that educates about the importance of organ donation, which they will share with their parents and talk about what they learned.

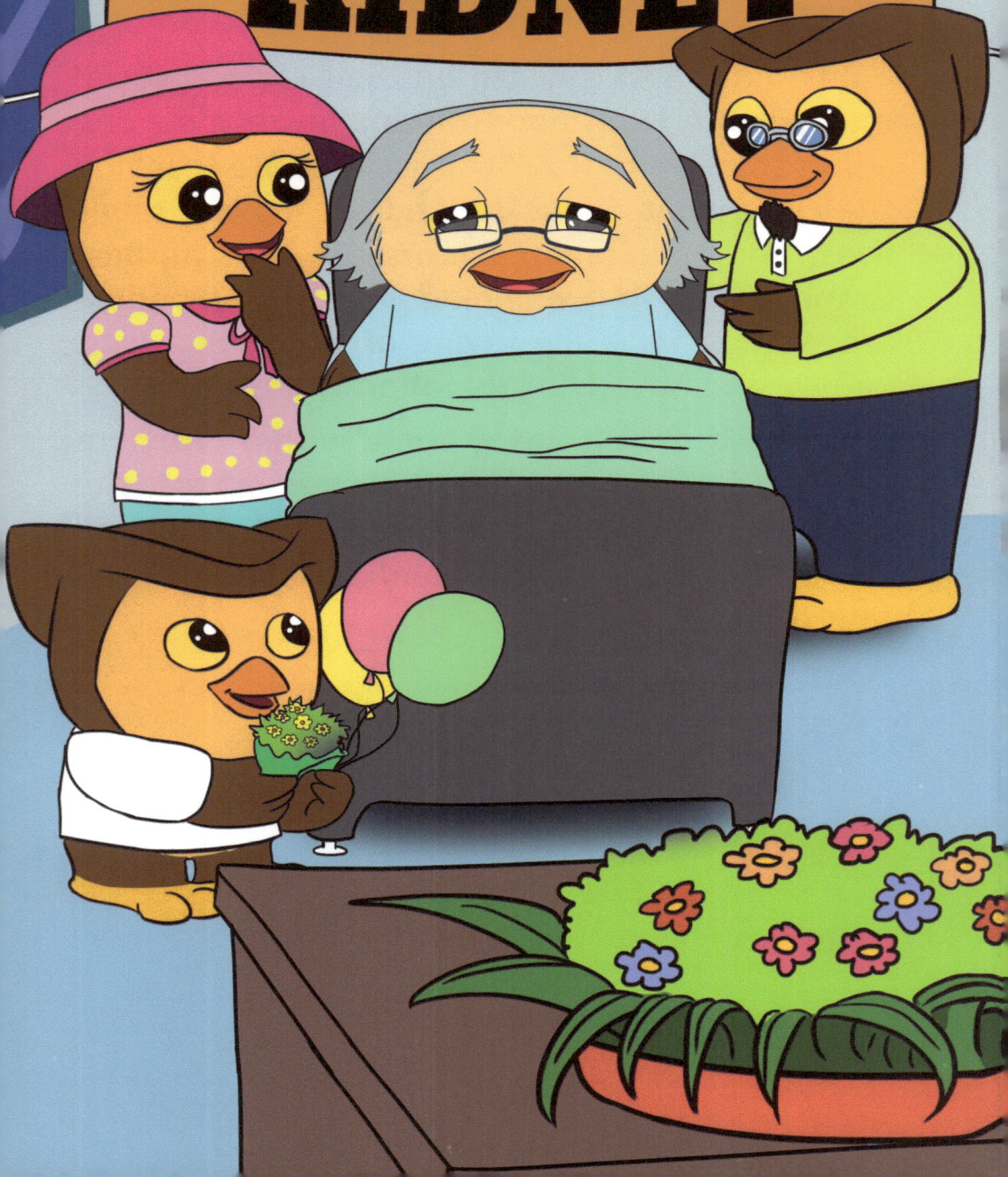

CONGRATS
NEW
on your
KIDNEY

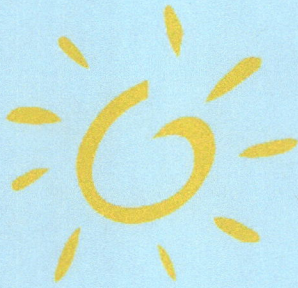

Four months after Howl visited the dialysis center to learn about the dialysis procedure, a kidney donor hero saved his Grandpa Bob! Howl and his family are so happy that this wonderful owl chose to donate his kidneys, and that the family honored those wishes.

Although dialysis helps keep you alive it can be strenuous on the body and time consuming. Howl's Grandpa Bob had been on dialysis for six years.

Howl and his family are grateful for the generous gift of life that helped save Grandpa Bob. They have written a letter to the donor family and will be meeting them in a few weeks at the Donor Remembrance Ceremony, where donor heroes and their families are honored for their wonderful gift to save someone's life.

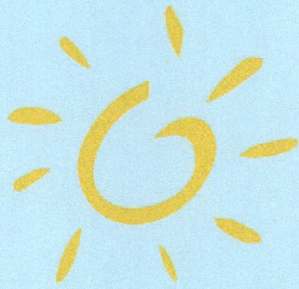

GLOSSARY

Blood Type – there are eight different possible types of blood in humans. These are A+, A-, B+, B-, AB+, AB-, O+, and O-

Chronic Kidney Disease – a disease that causes the kidneys to be sick and not do the job they are supposed to do

Dialysis – the process of filtering and removing excess water and harmful liquids from the human body when the kidneys cannot do this process naturally

Dialysis Technician – responsible for watching over the process of dialysis and operating the machines that assist in that process. The technician also monitors the patient during this time

Fistula – a special spot created by a surgeon (usually in the arm) connecting an artery to a vein, to create a stronger blood vessel

Hemodialysis – a treatment that removes wastes and extra fluids from the blood, which is pumped through soft tubes to a special machine where it is filtered outside of the body, and then returned to the bloodstream

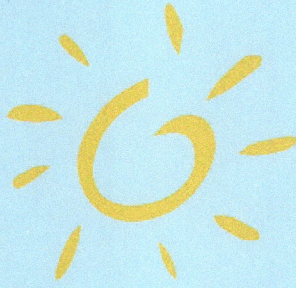

Kidney – the kidneys are a pair of bean-shaped organs on either side of your spine, below your ribs and behind your belly. Each kidney is roughly the size of a large fist. The kidneys' job is to filter your blood

Kidney Transplant – a surgical procedure to place a healthy kidney into a person whose kidneys no longer function properly

Organ Donation – a process of surgically removing an organ or tissue from one person, the organ donor, and placing it into another person, the recipient

Peritoneal Dialysis – a treatment where the blood is cleaned inside of the body, instead of outside

Transplant List – a list of people in the United States who are waiting for a life-saving organ

For information about dialysis, kidney health and transplant, please visit kidney.org (National Kidney Foundation), or donatelife.net

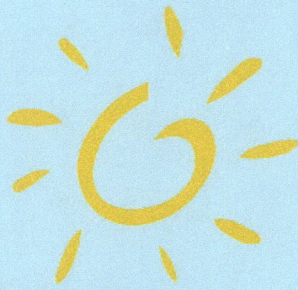

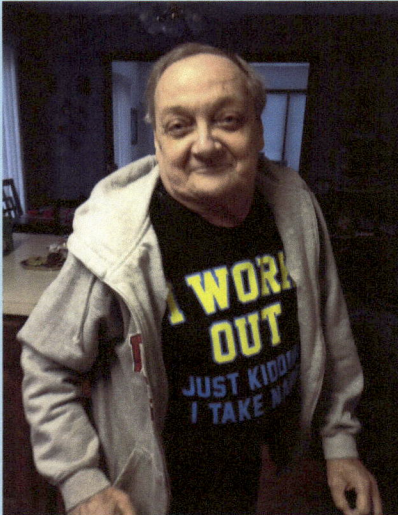

The real Grandpa Bob

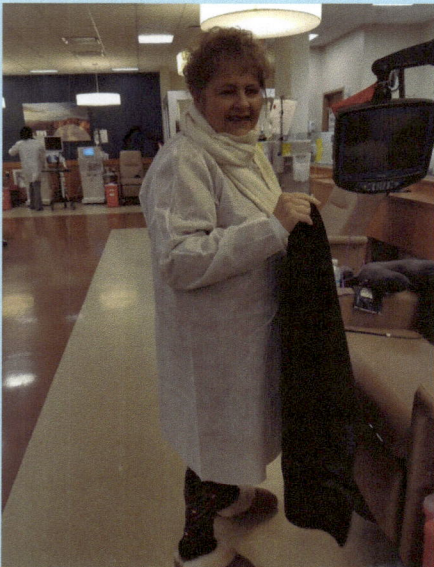

Pat Birrenkott

Pat and her technician
during dialysis treatment

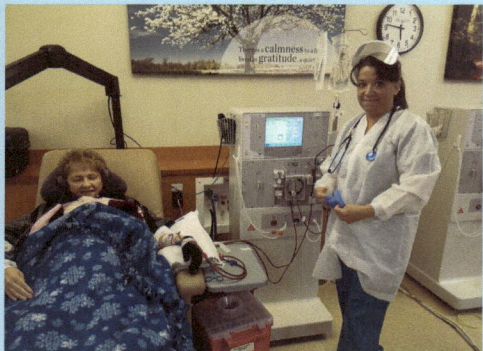

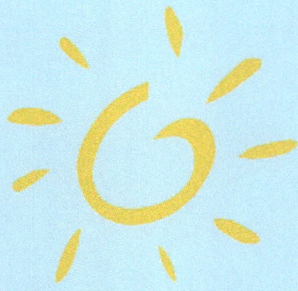

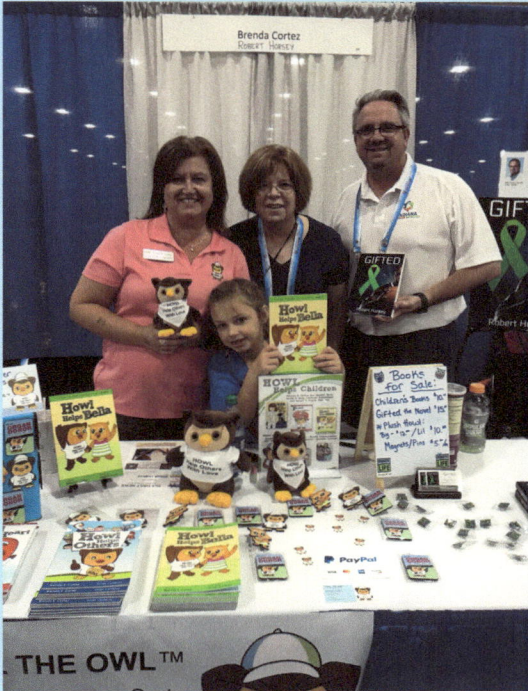

At the Transplant Games in Salt Lake City, Utah, with living kidney donor Lisa Hetzel, Robert Horsey, a recovery coordinator and author of the novel *Gifted*, and Bella-holding her book, *Howl Helps Bella*

My mom and me at the Nevada Network Donor Remembrance Ceremony

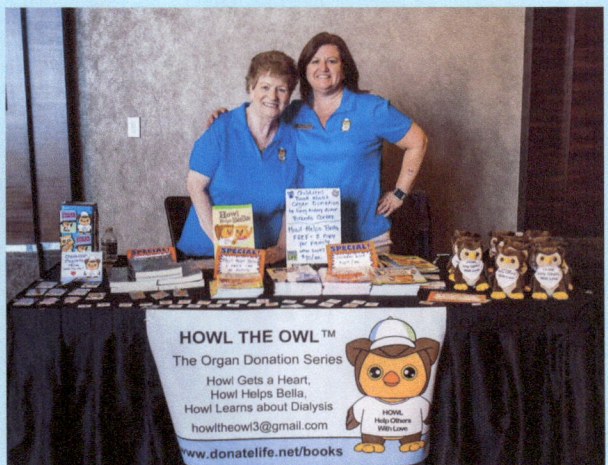

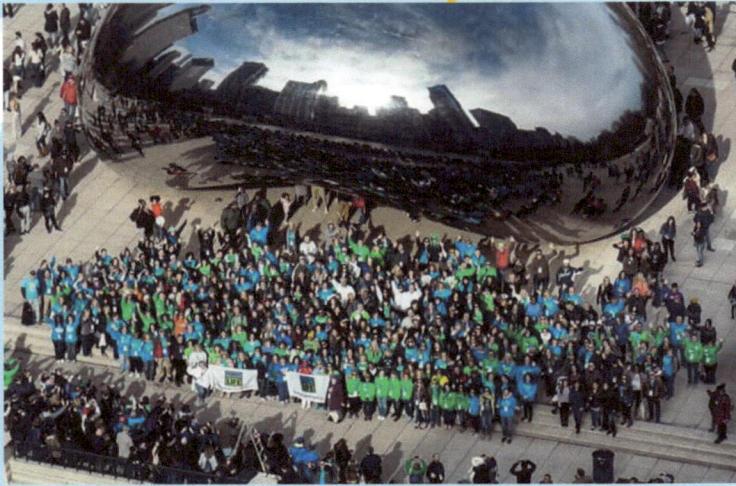

**2018 Living Donor Rally in Chicago
(photo by John F Martin)**

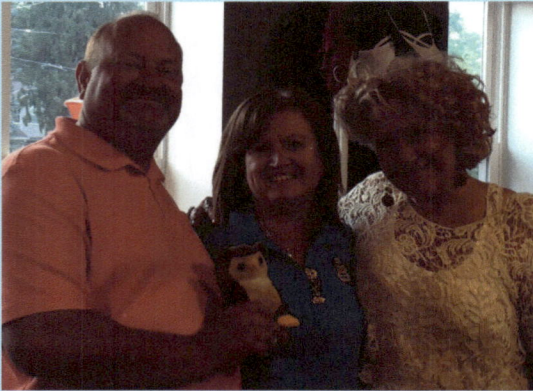

Kidney transplant
recipients Jeff Jacobsen
and Cindy with Howl
and me

My friend, publisher,
and living donor kidney
transplant recipient
Mike Nicloy

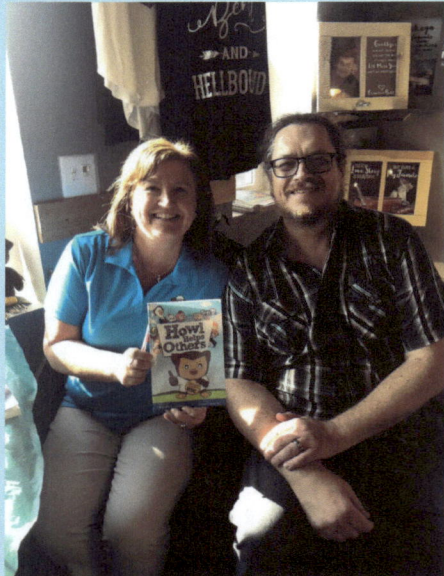

www.ingramcontent.com/pod-product-compliance
Lightning Source LLC
Chambersburg PA
CBHW041223270326
41933CB00001B/32